The RSD Advantage

A Practical Guide for ADHD Professionals to Stop Fearing Feedback and Turn Rejection Sensitivity into Your Professional Superpower

Ludwig Steven Cox

ISBN: 978-1-7641438-2-0
Isohan Publishing

The Silent Struggle of High-Achievers with ADHD

The blinking cursor on the screen seemed to mock Sarah. It had been ten minutes since her weekly check-in with her manager, Mark, and she hadn't typed a single word. Her heart was still hammering against her ribs, a frantic bird trapped in a cage. The project she had poured her last two weeks into—the one she was genuinely proud of—was now, in her mind, a complete and utter failure.

What had Mark actually said? He had leaned back in his chair, smiling, and said, "This is a great start, Sarah. The client is going to be pleased with the overall direction. Before we send it over, let's just refine the data visualization on slide five—it could be a bit clearer for the executive team."

He had said, **"great start."** He had said the client would be **"pleased."**

But what Sarah heard was entirely different. Her internal translator, an expert in distortion, had fed her this message instead: *You failed on slide five. Your work isn't clear enough. You're not thinking at an executive level. You almost embarrassed the team by sending this out. You are not good enough for this job.*

The physical sensation was immediate and overwhelming. A hot, prickly shame washed over her, starting in her chest and spreading to her fingertips. Her stomach churned. She felt a desperate urge to either run out of the building or to spend the next 72 hours perfecting that single slide to prove she wasn't an imposter. She avoided eye contact with her colleagues, certain they could see her incompetence written all over her face. This intense, painful, and hidden reaction is the daily reality for countless talented professionals with Attention-Deficit/Hyperactivity Disorder (ADHD).

The Problem

This is not simple sensitivity. It's not a lack of confidence or an inability to take feedback. This is **Rejection Sensitive Dysphoria (RSD)**, an extreme and painful emotional response to perceived or actual criticism, rejection, or failure. For those with ADHD, this experience is a near-constant companion in the workplace. It is an invisible storm that can rage internally while you present a calm, professional exterior.

This storm can sabotage your career in a hundred different ways.

- It can make you procrastinate on important projects because the fear of negative feedback is paralyzing.

- It can cause you to avoid speaking up in meetings, even when you have brilliant ideas.

- It can lead you to over-explain yourself or become defensive when a manager asks a simple question.

- It can make you ruminate for days—or weeks—over a minor comment, draining your mental energy and focus.

Many high-achievers with ADHD are masters of masking. You've likely developed complex systems to get by, to overcompensate for challenges with executive function, and to present a flawless front. But RSD is the crack in the armor.

It's the reason why, despite your intelligence and creativity, you may feel like you're always on the verge of being "found out."

The Promise

If Sarah's story feels familiar, know this: you are not alone, and you are not broken. This book is built on the firm belief that you can do more than just survive at work; you can build a career where you feel confident, secure, and valued. It offers a clear roadmap to transform your relationship with feedback and unlock the professional potential that RSD has held hostage.

We will not be offering vague suggestions or temporary fixes. We will give you a definitive framework for managing these intense emotions in the moment they happen. This is the **"Unrejected" framework**, a practical, three-step method:

1. **Acknowledge:** Recognize the physical and emotional signs of an RSD reaction as it begins, without judgment.

2. **Analyze:** Question the distorted narrative your brain is telling you and separate the facts of the feedback from the feelings of failure.

3. **Act:** Choose a deliberate, constructive action instead of reacting from a place of pain or fear.

This book will guide you through each step of this framework with concrete examples and tools. You will learn the science behind why you feel this way, identify your exact workplace triggers, and build a personalized toolkit to handle everything from a confusing Slack message to a formal performance review. Your sensitivity, once a source of pain, can become a source of great strength, empathy, and leadership. It's time to quiet the storm.

Chapter 1:The Brain Science of Rejection

The experience of rejection is universal. No one enjoys being criticized or left out. For most people, the sting of a negative comment is like a brief, sharp poke—unpleasant, but it fades quickly. For someone with ADHD and Rejection Sensitive Dysphoria, that same poke feels like a third-degree burn. The pain is not just more intense; it is fundamentally different in nature, searing and slow to heal.

To effectively manage these reactions, you first have to understand where they come from. Your intense feelings are not a personal failing or a character flaw. They are the result of your brain's unique wiring. This chapter will provide a straightforward explanation of RSD and the neurological reasons behind its powerful impact.

An Explanation of Rejection Sensitive Dysphoria

Rejection Sensitive Dysphoria is a term first popularized by Dr. William Dodson to describe an extreme emotional sensitivity and pain triggered by the perception—not necessarily the reality—of being rejected, teased, or criticized by important people[1] in your life [1]. It can also be triggered by a sense of failing to meet your own high standards or the expectations of others. "Dysphoria" is the Greek word for "unbearable," and that is a fitting description. When an RSD episode is triggered, the emotional pain is all-consuming and can feel physically unbearable.

It's helpful to distinguish RSD from other mood conditions.

- It is **not** a typical mood swing. The shifts are not random; they are always triggered by a perceived rejection or critique.

- It is **not** depression or anxiety, though it can certainly co-exist with them. The intense dysphoria of an RSD episode is often sudden and severe, but it can also pass just as quickly if the perception of rejection is relieved.

For professionals with ADHD, this can manifest as a sudden, catastrophic drop in mood. You might be having a productive, positive day, and a single email or comment can send you into an emotional tailspin, feeling worthless, ashamed, and deeply hurt. Because this happens internally, your colleagues and managers may have no idea of the turmoil you are experiencing. They only see the results: your sudden quietness, your defensiveness, or your avoidance of the next project.

The Emotional Sunburn Analogy

To make this more concrete, let's use an analogy. Think of emotional resilience as your skin's tolerance to the sun. Most people can spend some time in the sun without protection and be fine. They might get a little pink, but it doesn't ruin their day.

Now, imagine you have a severe **emotional sunburn**. Your emotional skin is raw, inflamed, and exquisitely sensitive. For you, even the gentlest touch—a suggestion from a colleague, a question from your boss—can cause a wave of intense pain. The "touch" itself isn't malicious, but your underlying condition makes it feel agonizing.

Mark's feedback to Sarah about her presentation slide was meant to be a gentle touch. But because of Sarah's emotional sunburn, it felt like a slap. Her reaction wasn't an overreaction to the feedback itself; it was a predictable reaction given her underlying neurological state. This is why telling someone with RSD to "toughen up" or "not take things so personally" is as useless as telling someone with a third-degree burn to just ignore the pain. The pain is real, and it has a biological basis.

The ADHD Brain on Rejection

So, what is happening in the brain to cause this "emotional sunburn"? While research is ongoing, current understanding points to the structure and function of the ADHD brain, particularly the interplay between a few key areas.

Think of your brain as having an alarm system and a control tower.

- **The Alarm System (The Limbic System, especially the Amygdala):** This is the primitive, emotional part of your brain. Its job is to scan for threats and, when it detects one, to sound the alarm. This triggers the "fight, flight, or freeze" response—pumping your body full of adrenaline and cortisol, raising your heart rate, and preparing you for danger.

- **The Control Tower (The Prefrontal Cortex):** This is the more evolved, rational part of your brain. It's responsible for executive functions like emotional regulation, impulse control, and logical reasoning. When the alarm goes off, the control tower's job is to assess the situation. Is this a real fire, or did someone just burn the toast? It's supposed to calm the alarm system down when the threat is not real.

In the ADHD brain, this communication system works a bit differently. Research, such as studies summarized by Dr. Russell A. Barkley, suggests that the prefrontal cortex—the control tower—is often under-activated and has weaker connections to the limbic system [2].

This creates a perfect storm for RSD.

1. **A Hypersensitive Alarm:** Your amygdala may be more likely to perceive social rejection as a threat on par with physical danger. A manager's neutral expression might be interpreted as a sign of anger.

2. **A Delayed Control Tower:** Your prefrontal cortex is slower to step in and say, "Hold on, let's assess this logically." It struggles to regulate the initial emotional blast from the alarm system.

The result? The fire alarm for "burnt toast" (a minor critique) sounds with the same deafening intensity as the alarm for a "house fire" (being fired). The emotional floodgates open, and the rational part of your brain is momentarily knocked offline, leaving you to drown in the feelings of shame and failure. This isn't your fault. It's neurology.

Self-Assessment: How Much Is RSD Impacting Your Career?

Now it's your turn to reflect. This quiz is not a diagnostic tool, but it will help you gauge the extent to which these experiences affect your professional life. For each question, choose the answer that best reflects your typical reaction.

1. A manager sends you a message that just says, "Can we talk for a few minutes this afternoon?" Your first immediate thought is:

a) "Great, I'm looking forward to connecting."

b) "I wonder what this is about. I'll prepare for a few different topics."

c) "Oh no. What did I do wrong? I'm in trouble."

2. You receive constructive criticism on a project you worked hard on. Afterward, you find yourself thinking about the negative parts for:

a) About an hour, then I move on.

b) Most of the day, but I can still focus on other work.

c) Days or even weeks; it's hard to think about anything else.

3. You speak up in a meeting, and no one immediately responds or acknowledges your point. You interpret this as:

a) People are processing what I said.

b) Maybe I should have explained it better.

c) That was a stupid idea. Everyone thinks I'm an idiot. I should never speak up again.

4. You notice a group of colleagues talking and laughing in the office. Your first instinct is to feel:

a) Happy that people are enjoying their day.

b) Curious about what they're discussing.

c) A pang of anxiety that they might be talking about you.

5. After a performance review that was 90% positive and 10% developmental feedback, you leave feeling:

a) Motivated and clear on my strengths and areas for growth.

b) Mostly good, but a little focused on the areas for improvement.

c) Devastated and completely focused on the 10% negative.

6. You make a small, correctable mistake at work (e.g., a typo in an internal email). Your level of internal shame is:

a) Low. I'll just correct it and move on.

b) Moderate. I feel a bit embarrassed but get over it.

c) High. I feel intense shame and worry about what people think of me.

7. How often do you avoid asking for help or clarification because you're afraid of "looking stupid"?

a) Rarely. I ask whenever I need to.

b) Sometimes, especially if I feel I should already know the answer.

c) Frequently. I'd rather struggle for hours than risk judgment.

8. How much energy do you spend trying to figure out what others are thinking of you at work?

a) Very little. I assume people will tell me if there's an issue.

b) A moderate amount. I try to be aware of social cues.

c) A huge amount. It's a constant background process in my mind.

Scoring Your Results:

- **Mostly A's:** RSD likely has a low impact on your work life. You have a naturally resilient response to feedback.

- **Mostly B's:** RSD may be moderately impacting your career. You experience the sting of rejection but have some ability to regulate it. The tools in this book can help you move more of your answers into the "A" category.

- **Mostly C's:** RSD is likely having a high impact on your professional life. The experiences described in this chapter are a regular, painful part of your reality. You are in exactly the right place.

Key Takeaways for this section

- Your intense emotional reactions to perceived criticism are not a character flaw; they are a real neurological phenomenon known as Rejection Sensitive Dysphoria (RSD).

- The "emotional sunburn" analogy helps explain why even minor feedback can feel intensely painful.

- RSD is linked to the ADHD brain's structure, specifically the interaction between a hypersensitive "alarm system" (the amygdala) and an under-regulated "control tower" (the prefrontal cortex).

- Understanding the "why" behind your reactions is the first and most necessary step toward taking control and managing them effectively.

With this foundational knowledge in place, you are no longer operating in the dark. You can now move from simply experiencing these reactions to actively investigating them.

The next chapter will turn you into a detective, helping you identify the specific clues and patterns that signal an RSD episode at work.

Chapter 2: Your Personal RSD Fingerprint

Identifying Your Triggers at Work

If RSD is the invisible storm, then triggers are the dark clouds that gather on the horizon, signaling its approach. A trigger is any specific event, interaction, or situation that sets off an RSD episode. For one person, it might be a manager's tone of voice; for another, it's the silence after they pitch an idea. These triggers are not universal; they are deeply personal. They form your unique "RSD Fingerprint."

Simply knowing that you have RSD is not enough. To effectively use the **Acknowledge, Analyze, Act** framework, you must first become an expert in your own triggers. Why? Because you cannot prepare for a storm you do not see coming. Awareness is your new superpower. It transforms you from a passive victim of your emotions into an active strategist. This chapter is a practical, hands-on workshop designed to help you map out your personal RSD fingerprint. Get a pen and paper or open a new document. It's time to gather some data.

Moving from Vague Anxiety to Specific Data

Most professionals with ADHD and RSD live with a constant, low-grade hum of anxiety. It's a feeling of "waiting for the other shoe to drop." This is mentally exhausting. The goal of this chapter is to replace that vague dread with specific knowledge. Instead of feeling a general sense of unease all day, you will be able to say, "I am heading into a 2 PM project review with David. This is a potential trigger situation for me. I need to have my plan ready." That shift is a game-changer.

We will do this by creating a **Trigger Log**. For the next week, your job is to be a detective of your own experiences. Your mission is to notice and note every time you feel that familiar, painful pang of rejection, shame, or failure. Don't judge it. Just log it.

Here is a simple structure for your Trigger Log:

1. **Date/Time:** When did it happen?

2. **The Situation:** What was the objective event? (e.g., "I sent an email to a client." "My manager asked me a question.")

3. **The Feeling:** What was the immediate emotional response? (e.g., "Sudden panic," "A wave of shame," "Crushing disappointment.")

4. **The Trigger Thought:** What was the exact thought that sparked the feeling? (e.g., "They'll think this is unprofessional." "He thinks my work is sloppy.")

Let's look at a case example.

Case Example: Maria's Trigger Log

Maria is a talented software engineer with ADHD who struggles with intense self-doubt. She decides to keep a Trigger Log for a few days.

Log Entry 1:

- **Date/Time:** Monday, 10:15 AM

- **The Situation:** My team lead, Ben, sent a Slack message: "Can you swing by my desk when you have a sec?"

- **The Feeling:** A jolt of pure fear. My stomach dropped.

14

- **The Trigger Thought:** "He found a major bug in my code. He's going to take me off the project. I'm going to be fired."

(What actually happened: Ben wanted to ask Maria for her opinion on a new software tool he was considering.)

Log Entry 2:

- **Date/Time:** Tuesday, 2:30 PM
- **The Situation:** I was in a team meeting and presented my idea for a new feature. After I finished speaking, there were a few seconds of silence before someone else spoke.
- **The Feeling:** Humiliation. I felt my face get hot.
- **The Trigger Thought:** "That was a terrible idea. Everyone knows it. I sounded like an idiot."

(What actually happened: The team members were thinking about her suggestion and how to best integrate it.)

Log Entry 3:

- **Date/Time:** Wednesday, 4:00 PM
- **The Situation:** I saw two senior engineers from another team talking near the coffee machine. They glanced in my direction and then laughed.
- **The Feeling:** Intense anxiety and paranoia.
- **The Trigger Thought:** "They're laughing at me. They must be talking about the mistake I made last week."

(What actually happened: They were laughing at a joke one of them told, and their glance in her direction was a coincidence.)

Maria's log already reveals a pattern. Her triggers are often ambiguous social cues: a vague message, a moment of silence, a glance from across the room. Her trigger thoughts immediately jump to the most negative possible conclusion. By simply writing this down, Maria has begun the process of separating objective reality from her subjective emotional reaction. This is the first step toward reclaiming her power.

Interactive Elements: Your Trigger Identification Checklists

Now, use the following checklists to help you pinpoint your own triggers. Go through them and check off any that resonate with you. Add any of your own that aren't on the list.

People-Based Triggers

These triggers relate to your interactions with specific individuals or groups.

- [ ] A manager or colleague with a very direct or blunt communication style.

- [ ] Someone with a flat or hard-to-read facial expression.

- [ ] Receiving feedback from a specific person you perceive as highly critical.

- [ ] Being interrupted or talked over in a meeting.

- [ ] Feeling ignored or left out of a conversation (in-person or online).

- [ ] Hearing a specific person's name in a negative context.

- [ ] A perceived change in someone's tone of voice (in-person or on the phone).

- [ ] Someone taking a long time to respond to your email or message.

- [ ] Not being invited to a meeting or social gathering you thought you should be a part of.

- [ ] Seeing people talking or laughing and assuming it's about you.

- [ ] *Your own addition:*
_____

- [ ] *Your own addition:*
_____

Task-Based Triggers

These triggers are related to the work you do and the processes around it.

- [ ] Starting a new or difficult project where you fear you might fail.

- [ ] Submitting work for review or approval.

- [ ] Receiving edits or tracked changes on a document you wrote.

- [ ] Presenting your work to a group.

- [ ] Getting a notification that a task you completed has been reopened or questioned.

- [ ] Being asked to estimate how long a task will take.

- [ ] Working on a task with unclear instructions or expectations.

- [ ] The moment right before a performance review.

- [ ] Being asked a question you don't immediately know the answer to.

- [ ] Realizing you've made a mistake.

- [ ] *Your own addition:*

  _____

- [ ] *Your own addition:*

  _____

Environment-Based Triggers

These triggers are connected to your physical or digital workspace and its culture.

- [ ] Vague, ambiguous communication via email or Slack/Teams. (e.g., "We need to talk," or a simple "?")

- [ ] A culture of sharp, "brutal" honesty or constant critique.

- [ ] An open-plan office where you feel constantly observed.

- [ ] A highly competitive environment where people are pitted against each other.

- [ ] Last-minute, urgent requests that throw you off your plan.

- [ ] The "ding" of a new email or message notification, bringing potential bad news.

- [ ] Company-wide announcements or reorganizations.

- [ ] Unstructured meetings with no clear agenda or facilitator.

- [ ] A general lack of positive feedback or recognition in the workplace.

- [ ] *Your own addition:*
  _____

- [ ] *Your own addition:*
  _____

By working through these lists and keeping your Trigger Log, you are building a detailed map of your personal RSD fingerprint. This is not an exercise in dwelling on the negative. It is an act of strategic intelligence gathering.

Key Takeaways for this section

- Your RSD triggers are unique to you and form your personal "RSD Fingerprint."

- The first step to managing RSD is to move from vague anxiety to a specific, data-driven awareness of your triggers.

- Keeping a **Trigger Log** is a definitive method for identifying the situations, feelings, and thoughts that precede an RSD episode.

- By categorizing your triggers as **people-based, task-based, or environment-based,** you can begin to see patterns and predict when you might be most vulnerable.

- This awareness is your new superpower. It allows you to prepare for challenging situations instead of being blindsided by them.

You have now done some of the hardest work. You've looked directly at the moments that cause you pain and started to catalog them without judgment. With this map in hand, you are now ready to learn the first-aid techniques you can apply in the heat of the moment. The next chapter will introduce the first step of our framework—Acknowledge—and provide a powerful technique to stop an RSD flare-up in its tracks.

A Concluding Reflection

The process of identifying one's own patterns of thought and feeling is not merely an intellectual exercise. It is a deeply personal form of inquiry that lays the groundwork for all meaningful change. By observing the self without immediate judgment, we begin to untangle the knots of automatic reaction that have constrained us. This act of careful self-observation is the first, and perhaps most profound, step toward self-regulation and, ultimately, self-acceptance.

Chapter 3: The "Name It to Tame It" Technique

Your First-Aid Kit for RSD Flare-Ups

You are in a meeting. Your manager turns to you and says, "I'm not sure this is the right direction for the project." Suddenly, the room feels ten degrees hotter. Your heart begins to pound a frantic rhythm against your ribs, and a thick fog of shame rolls into your mind. Your internal alarm is screaming, "FAILURE! DANGER! YOU ARE BEING REJECTED!" Every instinct tells you to either lash out defensively ("What do you mean? This is what we agreed on!") or to shrink into yourself, nodding silently while your mind spirals into a vortex of self-criticism.

This is the moment of choice. It is the precise point where you can either let the RSD storm take over or you can deploy your first-aid kit. The first and most necessary tool in this kit is a technique drawn from the work of neuropsychiatrist Dr. Daniel Siegel: **Name It to Tame It** [3]. The principle is simple: the act of applying a label to a strong emotional experience recruits the more logical, language-based parts of your brain, which in turn helps to calm the primitive, emotional parts that are firing on all cylinders. This chapter provides a step-by-step guide to using this technique and other immediate interventions to stop an emotional spiral before it takes over.

A Step-by-Step Guide to Recognizing the Onset

The RSD storm doesn't appear out of nowhere. Like a physical storm, it has warning signs. The key is to become a skilled meteorologist of your own internal weather. The flare-up begins with a physical cascade, often before you are even consciously aware of the emotional hit. Your first task is to learn to recognize these bodily signals.

Step 1: Notice the Physical Shift.

This is the first part of the Acknowledge phase of our framework. You must shift your focus from the external trigger (the words someone just said) to your own internal, physical state. Look for these common signs:

- A sudden hot or cold flush, often in the face, neck, or chest.

- A rapid increase in your heart rate.

- Shallow, quick breathing, or the sensation that you can't get enough air.

- A tightening or clenching in your stomach, chest, or throat.

- Suddenly tense muscles, especially in the shoulders, jaw, or hands.

- A feeling of dizziness or lightheadedness.

Case Example: Leo in the Boardroom

Leo, a marketing strategist, is presenting a new campaign concept. The Chief Financial Officer, a man known for his bluntness, interrupts him. "I don't see the ROI on this, Leo. It feels fluffy."

Immediately, Leo feels a hot flush creep up his neck. His stomach clenches into a tight, painful knot. His hands, holding the remote for the slides, feel clammy. In the past, he would have ignored these signals and pushed through, his voice getting tight and defensive. But now, he has a new plan. He pauses for a beat, takes a sip of water, and thinks to himself, *"Okay. There it is. Hot flush, clenched stomach. This is the start of an RSD episode."* He hasn't stopped the feeling, but he has noticed it. This is a huge victory.

Step 2: Name the Emotion.

Once you have identified the physical signal, give the emotion a name. This must be done internally, with a spirit of neutral observation—not judgment. You are not saying, "I am a failure." You are saying, "I am experiencing a feeling of intense shame." This simple shift in language creates a sliver of space between you and the emotion. You are the observer of the feeling, not the feeling itself.

Some labels you might use:

- "This is intense rejection."

- "This is a wave of shame."

- "This is the feeling of humiliation."

- "I am having a strong fear response."

Back in the boardroom, after noticing the physical signs, Leo's next internal thought is, *"Okay, and this feeling is intense humiliation."* He has now noticed the physical signs *and* labeled the emotion. He has successfully named it. Now, he can move to tame it.

Discreet Grounding Techniques for the Office

Naming the emotion is the first step in taming it. The next is to actively calm your nervous system. You need techniques that pull your brain's attention away from the internal storm and anchor it in the present, physical reality of the room.

Crucially, these must be things you can do at your desk or in a meeting without drawing any attention to yourself.

Here is your office-friendly grounding toolkit:

1. **The 5-4-3-2-1 Sensory Method (Abridged):** You can do this with your eyes open, looking at the person speaking to you.

   - **Subtly press your feet flat on the floor.** Feel the solid ground beneath you. Notice the texture of the carpet or the coolness of the tile through your shoes.

   - **Press your fingertips together.** Under the conference table or on your lap, gently press the pads of your fingers on one hand against the pads of your fingers on the other. Focus on the sensation of pressure.

   - **Feel the chair supporting you.** Notice the pressure of the chair against your back and legs. Feel its solidness.

   - **Find a neutral object to focus on.** Let your eyes rest on a pen, a glass of water, or the grain of wood on the table. Simply notice its color, shape, and texture without judgment.

2. **The Box Breathing Technique:** This is a powerful and completely silent way to regulate your breathing and heart rate. No one will know you are doing it.

   - Silently inhale through your nose for a count of **four**.

   - Hold your breath for a count of **four**.

- Silently exhale through your mouth for a count of **four**.

- Hold the exhale for a count of **four**.

- Repeat this cycle three or four times. This deliberate pattern forces your breathing to slow and deepen, which sends a signal to your brain that the danger has passed.

3. **Discreet Sensory Tools:** Many professionals with ADHD find that a small, discreet sensory object can be a powerful anchor.

   - **A smooth stone or "worry stone" in your pocket.** The cool, smooth texture can be very calming to rub with your thumb.

   - **A textured ring.** A ring with a spinning band or a bumpy texture allows you to give your fingers a task, channeling nervous energy.

   - **A small piece of putty or a stress ball.** You can squeeze this in your hand under a table or in your pocket.

Leo, standing in front of the CFO, begins the box breathing technique. As he listens to the critique, he inhales...two...three...four. He holds...two...three...four. He exhales...two...three...four. He also presses his feet firmly into the floor, feeling the anchor of the ground beneath him. The wave of humiliation is still there, but it's no longer a tsunami threatening to pull him under. He has created just enough mental space to think.

Scripts for "Buying Time" in a Conversation

You have named the emotion. You have used a grounding technique. Now you need one more tool: an exit ramp. You need to give yourself permission and time to process the feedback away from the intense pressure of the immediate moment. This is not avoidance; it is a strategic retreat. You need a few professional, polished, all-purpose phrases to create this space.

Here are your scripts. Memorize one or two that feel natural to you.

For direct feedback in a conversation:

- "Thank you for that feedback. I'd like to take a moment to process it and get back to you." (This is direct, professional, and clear.)

- "That's a helpful point. To make sure I address it properly, let me review my notes after this and I'll circle back this afternoon." (This shows you are taking it seriously.)

- "I appreciate you bringing this to my attention. I want to give this the thought it deserves. Can I follow up with you over email later today?" (This provides a different format for the follow-up, which can be less intimidating.)

When you are asked a question you can't answer:

- "That's a great question. I want to give you the most accurate information, so let me confirm that and get right back to you." (This reframes "I don't know" as "I am committed to accuracy.")

In the boardroom, Leo has used his grounding techniques. The CFO finishes his critique. Instead of becoming defensive, Leo uses a script. He says calmly, "Thank you for that perspective. The ROI is a critical point. Let me take another look at the projections with your feedback in mind and I will come back to you this afternoon with a revised approach."

He sounds confident. He sounds professional. He sounds like he is in control. Inside, his heart is still beating faster than normal, but he has successfully navigated the moment without letting the RSD storm dictate his response. He has bought himself time.

Key Takeaways for this section

- You can interrupt an RSD emotional spiral by using the **Name It to Tame It** technique, which involves recognizing the physical signs and then applying a label to the emotion.

- Discreet, office-friendly **grounding techniques** (like box breathing or focusing on sensory input) are essential tools for calming your nervous system in the heat of the moment.

- Having professional **"buying time" scripts** memorized is a definitive way to create the space you need to process feedback without reacting defensively.

- The goal is not to eliminate the initial feeling of pain, but to stop that feeling from hijacking your behavior. You can feel the sting of rejection and still act with poise and professionalism.

This is your first-aid kit. It is designed for immediate, in-the-moment care. But first aid is not a long-term cure. Now that you have created some space, the next step is to use that space wisely. The following chapter will teach you how to deconstruct and analyze the feedback you've received, so you can separate the facts from the feelings.

Chapter 4: The Pause and a Plan

Deconstructing Perceived Criticism

You did it. You used a "buying time" script and successfully exited the high-pressure situation. You've made it back to the relative safety of your desk or a quiet hallway. The immediate threat has passed, but the emotional residue of the RSD flare-up—that lingering feeling of shame or failure—is likely still present. This is a dangerous moment. It's the time when you might be tempted to ruminate, catastrophize, or jump to conclusions.

This is where the second stage of our framework, **Analyze**, comes in. The pause you created is useless unless you have a plan for how to use it. You need a structured way to deconstruct what just happened so you can respond logically instead of emotionally. We will use a simple, memorable framework for this analysis: **The 3 C's—Clarify, Categorize, and Choose.** This method will turn you from a passive recipient of criticism into an active investigator of information.

The 3 C's Framework for Analyzing Feedback

Your brain, in the throes of an RSD reaction, is an unreliable narrator. It takes ambiguous data and weaves it into a story of your own incompetence. The 3 C's framework is a tool for fact-checking that story.

First C: Clarify

Vague feedback is the natural enemy of someone with RSD. A comment like "This needs more polish" or "I'm just not feeling it" is an open invitation for your brain to fill in the blanks with its worst fears. "More polish" becomes "This is sloppy and unprofessional." "I'm not feeling it" becomes "This is a terrible idea and I have bad instincts." The first step in your analysis is to refuse to play this guessing game. You must get more specific information.

Of course, this often means going back to the person who gave the feedback—a daunting task. But you can do it without appearing defensive or needy. The key is to frame your questions as a good-faith effort to understand and implement their suggestions effectively. Your tone should be one of curiosity and collaboration.

Scripts for Asking Clarifying Questions:

- **For vague adjectives (e.g., "better," "stronger," "cleaner"):** "Thanks again for the feedback earlier. To make sure I'm on the right track, could you give me an example of what a 'stronger' version of this would look like to you?"

- **To narrow the scope:** "You mentioned the report needs some work. Could you point me to the specific section or data point you'd like me to revisit? It will help me focus my revisions."

- **To understand the underlying concern:** "When you said the campaign felt 'fluffy,' it was a helpful flag for me. Are you most concerned about the budget, the messaging, or the expected outcomes?"

Case Example: Leo Clarifies

Leo used his script to buy time from the CFO. He spent ten minutes at his desk using his grounding techniques until he felt his nervous system settle. Now, he knows he needs to clarify. He can't fix "fluffy." He drafts a brief email:

Subject: Following up on the campaign concept

Hi [CFO's Name],

Thank you again for your feedback in the meeting. I want to make sure I fully address your concerns about the ROI.

To help me focus my revisions, could you clarify which part of the plan felt 'fluffy'? Are you most concerned with:

1. *The projected ad spend?*

2. *The messaging and its connection to sales?*

3. *The way we plan to measure the results?*

Your guidance here will be a big help. I'm confident we can get this to a place you're happy with.

Best,

Leo

This email is brilliant for several reasons. It's professional. It shows Leo is proactive and takes feedback seriously. Most importantly, it forces a specific answer and takes the guesswork—and the emotional spiraling—out of the equation.

Second C: Categorize

Once you have clear feedback, you need to sort it. Not all feedback is the same, and it shouldn't all be treated with the same emotional weight. Sorting the feedback helps you to depersonalize it.

Ask yourself: What is this feedback *really* about?

1. **Is it about THE WORK?** This is feedback about a task, a document, a project, or a deliverable. Examples:

"This slide needs a clearer chart." "There's a calculation error in this spreadsheet." "This report needs a summary at the beginning." This is the most common and least personal type of feedback. It is not about *you*; it is about a *thing*. You can fix a thing.

2. **Is it about YOUR BEHAVIOR?** This is feedback about how you conduct yourself in the workplace. Examples: "You've been late to the last few team meetings." "You interrupted Sarah several times during her presentation." "When you get stressed, your emails can come across as abrupt." This feedback feels more personal and can sting more. It requires honest self-reflection.

3. **Is it a MISUNDERSTANDING?** Sometimes, feedback is based on incorrect information. Examples: "You missed the deadline on the Miller report" (but the deadline was moved). "You didn't include the Q3 data" (but you were told to use Q2 data).

After you've placed the feedback into one of these categories, you must ask one more critical question: **Is it valid?** Your RSD will tell you that all negative feedback is 100% true and a reflection of your deepest flaws. Your logical brain must act as a filter.

- **Consider the source:** Is the person giving the feedback generally a reasonable, constructive person? Or do they have a reputation for being overly critical or unclear?

- **Look for patterns:** Is this something you've heard from more than one person? If your manager and a colleague have both mentioned that your emails can be blunt, that's a valid data point to consider. If only one person who you have a difficult relationship with says it, it may be less about you and more about them.

- **Is it actionable?** "I don't like the color blue" is not actionable feedback. "We should use the company's official brand color blue" is. Valid feedback gives you a clear path forward.

Third C: Choose

This is the final and most empowering step of the analysis. Based on your categorization, you get to **choose** what to do next. You are in control.

1. **Choose to ACT.** If the feedback was about the work, was valid, and is now clear, the choice is simple: make a plan to act on it. Break it down into small, concrete steps. This moves you out of feeling and into doing, which is a powerful antidote to shame.

2. **Choose to REFLECT.** If the feedback was about your behavior and you've determined it's valid, the choice is to reflect. You might not have an immediate action item, but you can choose to be more mindful of that behavior going forward. You might say to yourself, "Okay, I will make a conscious effort to let others finish their thoughts in meetings."

3. **Choose to CORRECT.** If the feedback was based on a misunderstanding, your choice is to professionally correct the record. "Actually, my understanding was that the deadline was moved to Friday. Can you confirm that?"

4. **Choose to LET IT GO.** This is a perfectly acceptable choice. If you have analyzed the feedback and determined it is not valid, not actionable, or a reflection of the other person's issues, you can consciously choose to release it. You do not have to accept every piece of criticism that comes your way. Visualize putting the comment into a box, closing the lid, and placing it on a shelf. It is not yours to carry.

Key Takeaways for this section

- After creating a pause, you must use a structured plan to analyze what happened. The **3 C's framework—Clarify, Categorize, and Choose—**is that plan.

- **Clarify** by asking specific, non-defensive questions to turn vague criticism into actionable information. Refuse to fill in the blanks with your own negative assumptions.

- **Categorize** the feedback to depersonalize it. Is it about the work, your behavior, or a misunderstanding? Then, ask if it's valid.

- **Choose** your response. You can act on it, reflect on it, correct the record, or consciously decide to let it go. You are in control of how you respond to feedback.

By systematically deconstructing criticism, you rob it of its emotional power. You turn a painful, personal attack into a set of neutral data points that you can manage. This skill is foundational. But what if you could reduce the number of painful feedback moments in the first place? The next chapter will show you how

Chapter 5: The Art of a Graceful Conversation

Communicating Your Needs Without Oversharing

So far, we have focused on reactive strategies—what to do when an RSD trigger has already been pulled. These are your essential first-aid and analytical skills. Now, we shift to a proactive approach. How can you shape your work environment and interactions to minimize the likelihood of triggering RSD episodes in the first place? The answer lies in learning how to communicate your needs and preferences clearly, professionally, and gracefully.

Many people with ADHD hesitate to do this because of a deep-seated fear. You may worry that expressing your needs will make you seem "difficult," "demanding," or like you are "making excuses" for your ADHD. This chapter will provide you with the strategies and scripts to do this in a way that is not only safe but actually enhances your professional reputation. You will learn to frame your needs not as a list of demands, but as a proactive effort to produce your best work and be a more effective team member.

The Reframe: From "Difficult" to "Professionally Self-Aware"

Let's address the core fear head-on. The fear of being seen as difficult is a powerful deterrent. But it's based on a faulty premise.

- **The Fearful Premise:** "If I ask for what I need, my manager will think I'm high-maintenance and can't handle my job."

- **The Professional Reframe:** "A manager's job is to get the best performance out of their team. By clearly and respectfully communicating how I work best, I am helping my manager do their job. It shows that I am self-aware and invested in producing high-quality work."

Good managers do not want to guess. They appreciate clarity. Telling a manager, "I work best when I get feedback in writing," is infinitely more helpful than letting them guess, giving you feedback verbally, watching you get flustered, and then seeing your performance dip. Proactive communication prevents problems for everyone. You are not making excuses; you are providing a user manual for your own success. And you can do this without ever mentioning ADHD or RSD.

Strategies for Professional Communication

The key is to focus the conversation on the **work** and the **outcomes**, not on your personal feelings or diagnosis. Your manager doesn't need to know *why* vague feedback sends you into a spiral. They only need to know that *specific* feedback helps you produce better results faster.

General Principles:

1. **Time it right.** Don't have these conversations in the middle of a crisis or right after receiving negative feedback. The best time is during a calm period, like a regular one-on-one meeting or when starting a new project.

2. **Keep it positive and forward-looking.** Frame your needs in terms of what helps you succeed, not what

you dislike. Use "I work best when..." instead of "I hate it when..."

3. **Make it a two-way street.** Ask about your manager's communication style as well. This frames the conversation as a collaborative effort to find the best way to work together.

4. **Be specific and concise.** Don't present a long list of demands. Start with one or two key preferences that would make the biggest difference.

Scripts for Discussing Your Work Style and Feedback Preferences

Here are concrete scripts you can adapt. Read them aloud. Find the language that feels most comfortable for you.

Scenario 1: Starting with a New Manager

This is the ideal time to set the stage. During one of your initial meetings, you can say:

- "I'm really looking forward to working with you. As we get started, I find it's always helpful to chat briefly about work styles to make sure we communicate well. For my part, I've found I do my absolute best work when I have a clear sense of the priorities and deadlines for a project. I'm also someone who really thrives on specific feedback—it helps me learn quickly and make sure I'm aligning with your vision. How do you prefer to communicate and give feedback?"

Scenario 2: Requesting Clearer Agendas or Instructions

If you find that meetings are unstructured or project kick-offs are vague (both common RSD triggers), you can say:

- "To make sure I'm always fully prepared for our check-ins, I'd find it super helpful if we could use a brief, shared agenda. Even just a few bullet points sent out beforehand would be great for helping me organize my thoughts."

- "As we kick off this next project, would it be possible to get the main objectives and deliverables in a brief email? Having something written to refer back to really helps me stay on track and ensure I don't miss anything."

Scenario 3: Shaping How You Receive Feedback

This is often the most important conversation. You have options here, depending on what works best for you.

- **To request written feedback:** "I've learned over time that I'm able to process and act on feedback most effectively when I can see it in writing first. It gives me a moment to digest it. For bigger projects, would you be open to sending your main points in an email before we meet to discuss them? I find it leads to a much more productive conversation."

- **To encourage more positive feedback (to balance the negative):** "It's really helpful for my development to know what's working well in addition to what can be improved. Knowing what I should *keep* doing is just as important as knowing what I should change."

- **To ask for immediacy:** "If you see something that isn't quite right, please feel free to tell me right away. I much prefer getting small course-corrections in the moment rather than having things build up."

Case Example: Sarah's Graceful Conversation

Let's return to Sarah from the introduction. After a few weeks of using her RSD first-aid kit and the 3 C's, she feels ready to have a proactive conversation with her manager, Mark. She asks for a few minutes at the end of their regular one-on-one.

Sarah: "Mark, I wanted to chat for a minute about work style. I've been thinking a lot about what helps me do my best work for the team."

Mark: "Sure, sounds good."

Sarah: "I really appreciate the feedback you give me. I've realized that I'm able to use it most effectively when I have a little bit of time to process it before I have to respond. In the future, especially for bigger things like that presentation a few weeks ago, I would find it immensely helpful if you could send me your thoughts in a few bullet points ahead of our chat. It helps me come to the conversation prepared to ask good questions."

Mark: "Oh, sure. I can absolutely do that. That makes sense. I just want to make sure you're getting what you need to grow. If written notes help, that's an easy change for me to make."

Notice what Sarah did. She didn't say, "Your verbal feedback makes me spiral into shame." She framed it around her effectiveness ("use it most effectively") and her preparation ("come to the conversation prepared"). She made it an easy, reasonable request that helps Mark be a better manager to her. This is not being difficult. This is being a professional partner.

Key Takeaways for this section

- You can proactively shape your work environment to minimize RSD triggers by communicating your needs clearly and professionally.

- Reframe the conversation in your mind: you are not being "difficult," you are being a "professionally self-aware" partner who is invested in producing excellent work.

- Center your communication on work and outcomes, not personal feelings or diagnoses. Use positive, forward-looking language like "I work best when..."

- Use specific scripts to discuss your preferences around meeting agendas, project instructions, and—most importantly—how you receive feedback.

Final Thoughts

True self-advocacy in a professional setting is not a single, dramatic confrontation. It is a series of small, thoughtful conversations that build a foundation of mutual understanding and respect. It is the quiet, consistent effort to teach others how to bring out the best in you. This is not a sign of weakness that needs to be accommodated; it is a sign of strength and strategic self-management that ought to be admired. By engaging in these graceful conversations, you are not only caring for yourself—you are modeling a more effective and humane way of working for everyone around you.

Chapter 6: Mastering High-Stakes Conversations

Performance Reviews and Difficult Feedback

For many professionals with ADHD, the announcement of an upcoming performance review lands with the subtlety of a formal eviction notice. It can feel like a summons to stand trial for a year's worth of perceived inadequacies. This single event combines nearly every known RSD trigger: direct evaluation, potential for criticism, a formal power dynamic, and the high stakes of your compensation and career progression. The dread can be all-consuming, leading to weeks of anxiety beforehand and days of rumination afterward.

But it does not have to be this way. With the right preparation and a clear plan, you can transform this annual ordeal from a source of dread into a catalyst for genuine professional growth. This chapter is your dedicated guide to navigating the most triggering conversations at work. We will walk through a three-part strategy: a pre-review checklist to get you prepared, in-the-moment techniques to stay present and manage emotional flooding, and a post-review protocol to decompress and create a constructive action plan.

The Pre-Review Checklist: Preparing for Battle

You would not walk into a major exam without studying. Do not walk into your performance review unprepared. The work you do in the days leading up to the meeting is the most important factor in how it will unfold. Your goal is to arm yourself with data and to ground your mindset in reality, creating a powerful defense against the distortions of RSD.

1. **Gather Your Accomplishments (Your "Wins" File).**
   Your brain, especially under stress, has a powerful
   negativity bias. It will remember the one deadline you
   missed with painful clarity and completely forget the
   ten you met ahead of schedule. You must counteract
   this with objective data. In the week before your
   review, become an archeologist of your own success.
   Dig through your past year's work.

   o Review your calendar, sent emails, and
     completed project files.

   o List every project you completed.

   o Note specific, quantifiable results. Instead of
     "Improved the monthly report," write
     "Redesigned the monthly report, reducing
     generation time by 3 hours and receiving
     positive feedback from 3 department heads."

   o Include positive feedback you received from
     colleagues or clients. Print out the emails if
     you have to.

   o This is not bragging; it is creating an objective
     record to ground you when your emotions try
     to tell you a different story.

2. **Anticipate the Gaps (and Frame Them).** No one is a
   perfect employee. It is a near certainty that your
   manager will have some developmental feedback.
   Instead of waiting to be ambushed by it, anticipate it.
   Be ruthlessly honest with yourself in a low-stakes
   moment. Where did you struggle this year? What
   projects didn't go as planned?

- For each potential gap, frame it proactively. Instead of thinking, "I'm going to get hammered for being disorganized," you can prepare a statement like, "One area I'm focused on improving is my project management workflow. I've started using a new digital planner that is already helping me track milestones more effectively." This shows self-awareness and initiative, which turns a weakness into a strength.

3. **Set Your Mindset.** How you walk into the room matters. RSD wants you to walk in expecting a verdict. You must walk in with the mindset of a student or a scientist.

   - **Adopt a Mantra.** Choose a short phrase and repeat it to yourself before the meeting. Examples: *"This is data, not a judgment." "I am here to learn and grow." "My worth is not on the table."*

   - **Define Your Goal.** Your goal for the meeting is **not** to get a perfect score. Your goal is to **understand your manager's perspective** and **leave with a clear plan for the year ahead.** That's it. This is a much more achievable—and less terrifying—goal.

4. **Prepare Your Toolkit.** Bring the physical tools you'll need to stay grounded.

   - A notepad and pen. Taking notes is a powerful tool. It forces you to listen actively and gives your hands something to do.

- Your "Wins" file. You don't have to read it aloud, but having it with you is a powerful psychological anchor.

- A bottle of water. Taking a sip is a perfect way to create a natural pause.

- Your discreet grounding object (from Chapter 3).

During the Review: Staying Present in the Storm

The meeting has started. Your manager is talking. This is when your first-aid skills become paramount. Your primary job in this phase is to listen, absorb, and regulate.

- **Take Notes. Copiously.** Write down the specific words your manager is using. This serves two purposes. First, it keeps you focused on the external reality rather than your internal emotional spiral. Second, it gives you an accurate record to analyze later, free from emotional distortion. When your RSD-brain tries to tell you, "He said you were a complete failure," your notes will say, "He said there is an opportunity to improve client communication skills." These are very different things.

- **Breathe.** This is not a metaphor. Deliberately use the Box Breathing technique from Chapter 3. As your manager speaks, silently inhale...hold...exhale...hold. This will keep your nervous system out of "fight or flight" mode and allow your prefrontal cortex—your thinking brain—to stay online.

- **Clarify, Don't Defend.** When you hear criticism, your first instinct will be to defend yourself. Resist this urge. A defensive posture immediately shuts down the conversation. Instead, shift into clarification mode. Use the scripts from Chapter 4.

- ○ *Manager:* "I'd like to see you take more initiative on projects."

- ○ *Defensive You:* "But I do! I took the lead on the Acme project and no one helped me!"

- ○ **Strategic You:** "That's helpful feedback. Could you give me an example of a recent situation where you saw an opportunity for me to show more initiative? It would help me understand what to look for in the future."

- **Use Your "Buying Time" Scripts.** You are allowed to pause. If a piece of feedback is particularly stinging, it is perfectly acceptable to take a moment.

  - ○ "That's a really important point. Let me think about that for a second."

  - ○ Then, take a sip of water. Look at your notes. Take a full cycle of breath. This small pause can be the difference between an emotional reaction and a thoughtful response.

Post-Review: The Decompression Protocol and Action Plan

You survived. You walked out of the meeting. The immediate pressure is off, but the emotional hangover can be intense. What you do in the first few hours after the review is critical for your long-term well-being.

Step 1: The Mandatory Decompression. Do not go straight back to your desk and start ruminating over every word. You must give your nervous system a chance to reset.

- **Schedule a buffer.** Book the 30 minutes after your review as "busy" in your calendar.

- **Change your scenery.** Physically leave the office if you can. Go for a brisk walk around the block.

- **Change your sensory input.** Put on headphones and listen to music that makes you feel good. Buy yourself a coffee. Do something to engage your senses in a pleasant way and pull your mind out of the conversational loop.

- **Do not analyze the feedback yet.** Give yourself at least one hour—preferably more—of emotional distance before you even look at your notes.

Step 2: Create Your Action Plan. Later that day or the next morning, sit down with your notes. It is now time to use the **3 C's framework (Clarify, Categorize, Choose)** in a calm, controlled environment.

- Go through your notes and sort every piece of feedback.

- Create three lists on a piece of paper: **Act, Reflect,** and **Let Go**.

- For every item on the **Act** list, define a concrete, specific first step. "Be more proactive" becomes "Action Item: Propose a solution for the weekly reporting issue in the team meeting this Friday."

- For every item on the **Reflect** list, schedule time to think about it or talk it over with a trusted mentor.

- For every item on the **Let Go** list, consciously release it. Scribble it out, tear up the paper—do whatever helps you to formally discard it.

Case Example: Jamal's Review

Jamal, a data analyst, has his review on Thursday. On Monday, he creates a "Wins" document listing the three major dashboards he built and the positive feedback he got from the sales team. He anticipates his manager will mention his tendency to miss minor details in his reports when he's rushing. He prepares a response about a new double-checking process he's implementing. He walks into the review with the mantra, "This is data, not judgment."

During the meeting, he takes furious notes. When his manager brings up the detail-orientation issue, Jamal uses his prepared statement. His manager is impressed by his self-awareness. After the meeting, Jamal goes for a 20-minute walk while listening to a podcast. The next morning, he analyzes his notes. He puts "Improve detail-orientation" and "Get certified in new software" on his **Act** list. He puts "Contribute more in team brainstorming sessions" on his **Reflect** list. He puts his manager's offhand comment that he's "quiet" on the **Let Go** list, recognizing it wasn't actionable feedback. He leaves the process feeling not shamed, but empowered with a clear plan.

Key Takeaways for this section

- You can transform performance reviews from a source of dread into a catalyst for growth by using a structured, three-part strategy.

- A **pre-review checklist**—gathering wins, anticipating gaps, and setting your mindset—is the most effective way to prepare for a high-stakes conversation.

- **During the review**, your job is to use your full toolkit of grounding techniques, note-taking, and clarification scripts to stay present and avoid defensive reactions.

- A **post-review protocol** involving a mandatory decompression period followed by a structured action plan is essential for processing the feedback constructively.

Chapter 7: Building Your "Rejection Resilience" Muscle

From Self-Compassion to Strategic Risk-Taking

The tools and strategies we have discussed so far are immensely powerful for managing RSD episodes in the moment. They are your defense. But what about offense? How do you move beyond simply managing the pain of rejection and start to build a genuine, lasting resilience to it? How do you reduce the intensity of the "emotional sunburn" itself?

Resilience is not a trait you are born with. It is a skill you develop. It is a muscle that, like any other muscle, gets stronger with practice. This chapter will provide you with a workout plan for your resilience muscle. We will introduce the clinical concept of "gradual exposure" and adapt it for the workplace. We will then focus on the single most important element for sustaining this work: self-compassion, the definitive antidote to the harsh inner critic that fuels RSD.

The Theory of Gradual Exposure

In therapy, gradual exposure is a technique used to help people overcome phobias. If someone has a fear of spiders, a therapist doesn't start by putting them in a room full of tarantulas. They start small. First, they might look at a cartoon drawing of a spider. Then a photo. Then a video. Then they might look at a real spider in a sealed tank across the room. Each small, successful step desensitizes the nervous system's fear response. The brain learns, "This situation is uncomfortable, but I can survive it."

We can apply this exact same principle to the fear of rejection at work. Your goal is to intentionally expose yourself to a series of low-stakes situations that could result in minor rejection or criticism. Each time you take a small risk and survive—regardless of the outcome—you are teaching your brain that feedback is not a mortal threat.

Your Rejection Resilience Workout

This is a progressive program. Start at Level 1 and only move to the next level when you feel relatively comfortable. The point is to create a series of small wins.

Level 1: Micro-Risks (Building a Foundation)

The goal here is to get used to the simple act of putting yourself out there in a very small way.

- **Ask a trusted colleague for feedback on something trivial.** This is your starting point. Do not ask for feedback on your biggest project. Ask for feedback on something with almost no emotional stakes.

    - *"Hey, Sarah, can you look at this email subject line for me? Does it seem clear?"*

    - *"Jamal, which of these two chart colors is easier to read?"*

- **State a simple, low-stakes opinion in a meeting.** You don't have to present a groundbreaking idea. Just practice using your voice.

    - *"I agree with Maria's point about the deadline."*

    - *"Just to clarify, are we talking about the Q3 or Q4 numbers?"*

- **Send a "thank you" or "good job" message to a colleague.** This flexes the social-interaction muscle in a positive, low-risk way.

Level 2: Calculated Risks (Expanding Your Comfort Zone)

Once you've mastered the micro-risks, it's time to take slightly bigger—but still controlled—steps.

- **Volunteer for a low-stakes part of a presentation.** You don't have to do the whole thing. Offer to present the one or two slides you feel most confident about.

  - *"I can take the section on project background if that helps."*

- **Share a half-formed idea in a brainstorming session.** The purpose of brainstorming is to generate ideas, not to present perfect ones. Give yourself permission to share an idea that isn't fully baked.

  - *"This might be a bit out there, but what if we tried...?"*

- **Ask for feedback on a small but real piece of work.** Choose a small project or a single section of a larger one and ask a friendly manager or peer for their thoughts.

  - *"Mark, when you have a moment, could you glance over the first page of this report? I'd love to know if the tone is right before I write the rest."*

Level 3: Strategic Leaps (Approaching the Edge)

This level involves taking risks that feel genuinely challenging, but which have a high potential for growth.

- **Ask for feedback *outside* of a formal review cycle.**
  This is a power move. It shows you are proactive
  about your growth and it gives you practice receiving
  feedback in a less formal setting.
    - *"Hi Sarah, I'm really trying to improve my
      presentation skills this year. If you notice
      anything in today's meeting—good or bad—
      would you be open to sharing it with me
      afterward?"*

- **Pitch a "stretch" project or idea.** Propose something
  that you are not 100% sure how to execute but are
  passionate about. This is a risk that could lead to a
  huge reward.

- **Respectfully disagree with someone in a meeting.**
  This can be one of the most difficult things to do. It
  must be done professionally, but it is a definitive act
  of self-confidence.
    - *"I see your point about option A, but I have
      some concerns about the budget. Could we
      explore how option B might be more cost-
      effective?"*

With every one of these exercises, the outcome is not what
matters most. Getting positive feedback is great, but getting
constructive criticism—and surviving it using your tools—is
an even bigger win for your resilience muscle.

Self-Compassion: The Antidote to the Inner Critic

You cannot build resilience through brute force alone. The
engine of RSD is a viciously harsh inner critic. The only way
to silence that critic is to cultivate an inner voice that is

compassionate. Dr. Kristin Neff, a leading researcher on this topic, has identified three core components of self-compassion [4]. This is your new internal operating system.

1. Self-Kindness vs. Self-Judgment.

Self-kindness means treating yourself with the same care and concern you would show a good friend who was struggling. When a friend makes a mistake at work, you don't call them a worthless failure. You say, "That sounds so tough. It's okay, everyone makes mistakes. What can you do to fix it?" You must learn to direct this voice inward.

- o **Instead of:** "I can't believe I said that. I'm such an idiot."

- o **Try:** "Wow, that came out more awkwardly than I intended. That feels embarrassing. It's okay, social interactions can be hard sometimes."

2. Common Humanity vs. Isolation.

RSD thrives on the feeling of isolation—the belief that you are uniquely and fundamentally flawed. Common humanity is the recognition that suffering and personal inadequacy are part of the shared human experience. Everyone makes mistakes. Everyone feels embarrassed. Everyone gets rejected sometimes. You are not alone in this.

- o **Instead of:** "What is wrong with me? No one else struggles like this."

- o **Try:** "This is a really painful feeling, but it's a human feeling. Many people feel this way when they get criticized at work."

3. Mindfulness vs. Over-Identification.

Mindfulness means observing your negative thoughts and emotions without getting swept away by them. It is the opposite of over-identification, where you fuse with your feelings (I am a failure). This links directly back to our "Name It to Tame It" technique. You are acknowledging your pain without letting it define your reality.

> o **Instead of:** "This feeling of shame is the truth of who I am."
>
> o **Try:** "I am noticing a strong feeling of shame right now. It is a powerful feeling, but it is a feeling. It is not the entirety of who I am."

Practicing self-compassion is not a passive activity. It is an active and courageous choice to be on your own side, especially when you feel you have failed. It is the foundation upon which all true resilience is built.

Key Takeaways for this section

- Resilience is not a fixed trait; it is a skill that can be built through deliberate practice, like strengthening a muscle.

- **Gradual exposure**—taking a series of small, calculated risks in the workplace—is a definitive method for desensitizing your nervous system to the fear of rejection.

- A progressive **"resilience workout,"** moving from micro-risks to strategic leaps, allows you to build confidence through a series of small wins.

- **Self-compassion** is the essential antidote to the harsh inner critic of RSD. Practicing self-kindness, recognizing your common humanity, and mindfully observing your feelings are necessary for sustainable growth.

Chapter 8: Turning RSD Challenges into Career Strengths

For most of this book, we have treated Rejection Sensitive Dysphoria as a problem to be managed—a storm to be weathered, a fire to be put out. We have focused on defensive strategies and coping mechanisms. This work is necessary. But it is only half of the story. To truly thrive, you must move beyond simply neutralizing the negative and begin to recognize the powerful and unique strengths that are often the other side of the same coin.

Your ADHD brain is not a defective version of a "normal" brain. It is a different kind of brain, with a different set of operating instructions. The very wiring that makes you so exquisitely sensitive to rejection can also be the source of your greatest professional assets. This chapter is about reframing the narrative. It's time to stop seeing your sensitivity only as a liability and start seeing it as the foundation for a unique kind of genius.

The Power of Deep Empathy

The intense emotional attunement of RSD means you are highly sensitive to the social and emotional currents around you. When unmanaged, this feels like a curse. You absorb everyone's moods, you read negativity into a neutral expression, and you feel responsible for the emotional state of every room you enter.

But when you have learned to manage the painful parts of this sensitivity, what remains is an almost uncanny ability to understand people. This is **empathy**, and it is a workplace superpower.

- **As a leader:** Your intuitive grasp of your team's morale and individual struggles can make you an incredibly supportive and effective manager. You don't need to be told when someone is feeling overwhelmed or disengaged; you can feel it. This allows you to intervene with support and encouragement long before a small issue becomes a major problem.

- **As a colleague:** You are likely the person colleagues come to when they need to vent or seek advice, because they know you will truly listen and understand. This makes you a central, trusted hub in your team's social network.

- **In sales or client service:** Your ability to sense a client's unspoken concerns or true needs gives you a massive advantage. You can build rapport and trust quickly because clients feel that you genuinely "get" them.

Success Story: Maria, the Empathetic Project Manager

Maria, the engineer from Chapter 2, used to be terrified of team meetings. She would interpret every silent pause as a judgment on her ideas. After learning to manage her RSD, she began to reframe her sensitivity. She realized she could sense the team's confusion about a project plan long before anyone spoke up. Instead of internalizing this as "They think my plan is bad," she started seeing it as valuable data. She began to proactively say, "I'm sensing there might be some confusion around the timeline. Let's pause and walk through it again to make sure we're all on the same page." Her team started seeing her as an incredibly perceptive and considerate leader. Her sensitivity, once a source of private pain, became her leadership signature.

The Drive for Meticulous, High-Quality Work

The intense fear of being criticized for making a mistake can be paralyzing. It can lead to procrastination and perfectionism. However, once you have tools to manage the paralysis, the underlying drive doesn't disappear. Instead, it can be channeled into a powerful commitment to excellence.

Your desire to avoid the pain of negative feedback can make you:

- **Extraordinarily thorough:** You are likely to be the person who double- and triple-checks the data, who proofreads the report one last time, and who thinks through every possible contingency before a project launch.

- **Deeply prepared:** The fear of being asked a question you can't answer can motivate you to prepare for meetings and presentations with a level of depth and detail that others might skip.

- **Committed to quality:** You take immense pride in submitting work that is flawless, not just to avoid criticism, but because you have an internalized high standard for what constitutes "good" work.

This is not the same as perfectionism, which is often a paralyzing state. This is a healthy, productive drive for quality that is a huge asset to any team or organization.

The Justice-Driven Advocate

RSD is not just about the fear of personal rejection. It often comes with a heightened sensitivity to injustice, unfairness, and cruelty in all its forms. Seeing a colleague treated unfairly or a bad policy being implemented can trigger the same intense, painful dysphoria as a personal critique.

While painful, this justice sensitivity can make you a powerful and passionate advocate for a better workplace.

- You are often the first to notice when a team member is being excluded or when a process is creating an unfair burden on certain people.

- You are less likely to tolerate toxic behavior or unethical shortcuts.

- When you channel this passion constructively, you can become a moral compass for your team and a driving force for positive change.

Success Story: David, the Creative Problem-Solver

David worked in logistics and was constantly frustrated by inefficient systems that created stress for his team. His intense reaction to this "unfair" system used to manifest as angry complaints. After learning to manage his emotional reactions, he started channeling that same energy into finding solutions. He became obsessed with designing a better workflow. His non-linear, ADHD-style of thinking allowed him to see connections and possibilities that others had missed. He presented a detailed proposal to his leadership, not as a complaint, but as a well-researched business case. The company implemented his system, which saved thousands of dollars and dramatically improved team morale. His frustration, once a liability, became the engine of his greatest professional achievement.

Finding Your Own Advantage

Your unique combination of traits will give rise to your own specific advantages. Take some time to reflect on the "challenges" of your ADHD and RSD. For each one, ask yourself: What is the other side of this coin?

- If you have a tendency to **hyperfocus**, where can you aim that intense concentration to become the go-to expert on a subject?

- If you have a "busy brain" with a million ideas, how can you use that creativity to become an innovation engine for your team?

- If you are intensely curious, how can that drive you to ask the questions that lead to breakthroughs?

Your wiring is not a bug; it's a feature. It comes with challenges, certainly, but it also comes with a suite of strengths that the world desperately needs. The final step in managing RSD is to embrace these strengths and put them to work.

Key Takeaways for this section

- The very traits that make RSD challenging can also be the source of your greatest professional strengths when they are understood and managed.

- Your intense emotional sensitivity, when reframed, becomes **deep empathy**, a superpower in leadership, collaboration, and client relations.

- The drive to avoid the pain of criticism can be channeled into a productive commitment to **meticulous, high-quality work.**

- Your sensitivity to unfairness can make you a passionate and effective **advocate for a better, more equitable workplace.**

- By reframing your challenges as strengths, you can stop just surviving at work and start leveraging your unique wiring as a genuine career advantage.

Chapter 9: Creating ADHD-Friendly Workplaces

Throughout this book, our focus has been primarily on individual strategies—your personal toolkit for managing RSD and building resilience. This internal work is the foundation. But at some point, you may look up from your own efforts and realize that you are constantly swimming against the current. You may work in a culture or a system that is inherently difficult for a neurodivergent brain to navigate.

While you cannot single-handedly change an entire corporate culture, you can be a powerful catalyst for positive change. This chapter is about moving from individual coping to collective improvement. It is a guide to advocating for neurodiversity-affirming practices in a way that is professional, strategic, and beneficial for everyone—not just for those with ADHD. You will learn how to speak to leadership and HR not from a place of needing accommodation, but from a place of offering a better way of working for the entire organization.

The Shift from Accommodation to Universal Design

The traditional way of thinking about workplace support is through the lens of "accommodations." This is a reactive model where an individual discloses a disability and requests specific changes to help them do their job. While this is a legally protected and sometimes necessary path, it can feel isolating and stigmatizing.

A more powerful and inclusive approach is to advocate for practices based on the principles of **Universal Design**. The concept of Universal Design, originally from architecture, suggests that environments should be designed to be as accessible as possible to everyone, regardless of their age, ability, or status [5]. A ramp alongside a staircase, for example, helps people in wheelchairs, parents with strollers, and delivery workers with carts. It is a universal benefit.

In the workplace, this means advocating for changes that help people with ADHD but also make work easier and more efficient for the entire team. This is your strategic key. You are not asking for "special treatment." You are proposing smarter, clearer, more effective ways of working that will boost productivity and engagement for all.

How to Talk to HR and Leadership

Advocating for change can be intimidating. Here is a structured approach to make the conversation as productive as possible.

1. **Frame it as a Business Proposal, Not a Personal Complaint.** Leadership and HR are primarily concerned with organizational health, productivity, and retention. Frame your suggestions in this language.

   o **Instead of:** "The way we run meetings is chaotic and stressful for me."

   o **Try:** "I have some ideas on how we could refine our meeting structure to improve efficiency and ensure we get the most out of everyone's time."

2. **Come with Solutions, Not Just Problems.** Do not just point out what is broken. Propose a clear, simple, and actionable solution.

   - **Instead of:** "No one ever knows what's going on."

   - **Try:** "I think we could reduce confusion and save time by implementing a standard practice of sending a brief recap email with key decisions and action items after every project meeting. I've drafted a simple template we could use."

3. **Focus on Universal Benefits.** For every suggestion you make, be prepared to explain how it helps everyone.

   - *"Sending out an agenda before meetings helps people with processing differences to prepare, but it also helps everyone else to arrive focused and ready to contribute."*

   - *"Using a shared digital task board to track project progress reduces anxiety for those who fear things falling through the cracks, but it also gives the entire team and leadership a clear, real-time view of our workload and priorities."*

A Menu of ADHD-Friendly (and Just Plain Good) Practices to Advocate For

Here is a list of common-sense changes you can propose that create a more neuro-inclusive environment.

- **Communication Clarity:**

- The Rule of 3: For any important request, communicate it in three ways: verbally, in a follow-up email, and on a shared task list. This ensures clarity and provides a written record.

- **"Headlines First":** A culture where people start emails or messages with a clear subject line or a one-sentence summary of the key point, rather than a long, rambling preamble.

- **Meeting Rhythms:**

  - **Agendas are Mandatory:** A simple rule that no meeting is put on the calendar without at least 2-3 bullet points outlining the topics to be discussed.

  - **Clear Facilitation:** Having a designated facilitator for each meeting whose job is to keep the conversation on track and ensure everyone gets a chance to speak.

  - **Action-Oriented Recaps:** A standard practice of ending every meeting with a verbal recap of decisions and action items, followed by a brief written summary.

- **Feedback Culture:**

  - **Structured Feedback Models:** Advocate for training managers on simple models like the **Situation-Behavior-Impact (SBI)** model. Instead of "You're too quiet in meetings," feedback becomes "In the project meeting this morning (Situation), when we were brainstorming ideas (Behavior), you didn't speak up. The impact was that the team missed out on your perspective (Impact)." This is specific, objective, and non-judgmental.

- ○ **Separating Feedback from Compensation:** Suggesting that developmental conversations and salary conversations be held at different times of the year to reduce the fear and pressure associated with performance reviews.

- **Work Environment Flexibility:**

  - ○ **Focus Time Norms:** Promoting a culture where it's acceptable to block off "focus time" on calendars and to turn off notifications. Encouraging the use of status messages like "Heads down on the budget until 2 PM."

  - ○ **Multiple Ways to Contribute:** Creating systems where people can contribute ideas in different ways—not just by speaking up in a fast-paced meeting, but also by adding comments to a shared document beforehand or sending ideas in a follow-up email.

By advocating for these kinds of practices, you are acting as an architect of a better workplace. You are using your unique perspective to identify the cracks in the system and propose intelligent, elegant solutions that shore it up for everyone.

Key Takeaways for this section

- You can move from individual coping to creating systemic change by advocating for neurodiversity-affirming practices.

- Frame your advocacy around the principles of **Universal Design**, proposing solutions that benefit everyone, not just those with ADHD.

- When speaking to HR or leadership, approach it as a **business proposal**, focusing on benefits like productivity and retention, and coming with clear solutions.

- Advocate for specific, practical changes in communication, meeting structure, and feedback culture that create a clearer, more predictable, and more effective work environment for all.

Conclusion: Thriving, Not Just Surviving

We began this journey with the story of Sarah, a talented professional whose career was being silently sabotaged by the invisible storm of Rejection Sensitive Dysphoria. Her story of feeling intense shame from a minor critique is a familiar one for countless high-achievers with ADHD. The path from that moment of painful, isolating paralysis to a place of confidence and professional success can seem impossibly long.

But you now hold the map for that journey. This book has provided you with a definitive framework and a practical toolkit to navigate that path. You have learned that your intense reactions are not a character flaw, but a neurological reality. You now have the power to manage that reality.

A Recap of Your Framework

The **"Unrejected" framework** is your new operating system for handling feedback and criticism in the workplace. It is a simple, three-step process to fall back on when you feel the storm begin to gather.

1. **Acknowledge:** You learned to recognize the first physical signs of an RSD episode and to use the "Name It to Tame It" technique to create a crucial pause between feeling and reaction. You have a first-aid kit of grounding techniques and "buying time" scripts to keep you from being swept away.

2. **Analyze:** You learned how to use that pause wisely. With the **3 C's framework—Clarify, Categorize, and Choose**—you can now deconstruct criticism,

separate the facts from the feelings, and make a conscious choice about how to respond. You are no longer at the mercy of vague feedback or your own worst assumptions.

3. **Act:** You learned to move from a defensive, reactive posture to a proactive, strategic one. You have scripts to communicate your needs gracefully, a plan to master high-stakes conversations, and a workout to build your resilience muscle over time. You have even learned to reframe your challenges as advantages and to advocate for a better workplace for everyone.

Thriving Because of Your Wiring, Not in Spite of It

Managing RSD is not about erasing your sensitivity or becoming a hardened, unfeeling version of yourself. In fact, the journey of managing this trait is what builds the very skills that can make you an exceptional professional.

The work you have done to understand your triggers has given you a level of **self-awareness** that many people never achieve. The practice of calming your own emotional storms builds a profound **emotional regulation** capacity. The effort it takes to face feedback constructively builds true **resilience**. And the journey of learning self-compassion can unlock a deep well of **empathy** for others.

These are not just coping skills; these are leadership skills. The very process of taming your greatest challenge is what forges your greatest strengths.

This book was designed to be a practical guide. But more than that, it is an invitation. It is an invitation to redefine your professional narrative. You are not a "problem employee" who needs to be fixed. You are a creative, sensitive, and intelligent professional with a unique perspective to offer. You now have the tools to ensure that your voice is heard, your work is valued, and your potential is fully realized. The goal was never just to survive at work. It is, and always has been, to thrive.

A Final Thought on Practice

The insights and frameworks presented in these pages are not passive knowledge to be acquired, but active skills to be practiced. There will be days when you execute these strategies with grace and precision. There will be other days when you are caught off guard and an RSD storm hits with its full, unmitigated force. On those days, the most important practice of all will be the one detailed in Chapter 7: self-compassion. The goal is not perfection. It is progress. It is the commitment to return to these tools, to be kind to yourself when you falter, and to take the next small step forward. This path is not a straight line, but a spiral. Each time you revisit these practices, you do so from a place of greater strength and deeper self-awareness.

References

[1] Dodson, W. (2019). Rejection Sensitive Dysphoria: A Misunderstood Condition. ADDitude Magazine.

[2] Barkley, R. A. (2015). Attention-Deficit Hyperactivity Disorder: A Handbook for Diagnosis and Treatment (4th ed.). The Guilford Press.1

[3] Siegel, D. J. (2010). Mindsight: The New Science of Personal Transformation. Bantam Books.

[4] Neff, K. (2011). Self-Compassion: The Proven Power of Being Kind to Yourself. William Morrow.

[5] Center for Applied Special Technology (CAST). (2018). Universal Design for Learning Guidelines version 2.2. Retrieved from http://udlguidelines.cast.org

* 9 7 8 1 7 6 4 1 4 3 8 2 0 *